DENTAL MERCURY DETOX

BY

Sam Ziff
Michael F. Ziff, D.D.S.
Mats Hanson, Ph.D.

Bio Probe, Inc., Publisher
Orlando, Florida

Bio-Probe, Inc is publishing a series of Health Information Guides. Each book in the series will cover a different subject associated with the presence of silver/mercury dental material in the oral cavity and its toxic potential to affect health.

The Health Information Guide Series is dedicated to providing the public and health professionals with scientific information related to the title subject matter. It is not intended as medical advice. Its intention is solely informational and educational. Please consult a Dentist, Physician or other Health Professional should the need for one be warranted.

Published in the United States of America
by Bio-Probe, Inc
P.O. Box 608010
Orlando, FL 32860-8010

CONTENTS

INFORMATION ON MERCURY DETOXIFICATION

Dorland's Medical Dictionary defines metabolic detoxification as: "reduction of the toxic properties of a substance by chemical changes induced in the body, producing a compound which is less poisonous or is more readily eliminated."(1)

Your body's normal biochemical processes routinely detoxify many dangerous by-products of metabolism as well as foreign substances that enter the body that have no metabolic function. Mercury falls in the latter category as it is a poison for which no human requirement has ever been identified.

We are all subjected to mercury in our food, water and air. If we were not exposed to any other source of mercury, most of us would probably be able to routinely cope without experiencing any of the signs or symptoms of mercury toxicity. That is because nature has provided some hidden safeguards. For example, the largest source of dietary mercury is derived from fish. However, the National Academy of Sciences has also stated that "The most consistent beneficial influence of selenium has been a reduction of the lethal and neurotoxic effects of methylmercury compounds."(2) Scientists have demonstrated that fish with higher levels of methylmercury generally also contained even higher levels of selenium, and conclude that the methylmercury ingested under these conditions is less toxic than methylmercury ingested under other circumstances.(2) [This means that mercury from the diet (fish) is not as dangerous as inhaled mercury vapor from dental fillings.]

However, there is a large segment of our population, some estimate as many as 75%, that have a source of mercury implanted in their body. That source of chronic mercury vapor exposure is silver/mercury dental fillings (also called amalgam fillings). As long as you have silver/mercury dental fillings you will be inhaling mercury vapor 24 hours a day, 365 days a year. In fact, some of the world's leading experts on mercury toxicology have recently concluded that the release of mercury from dental amalgams is a major contributor to mercury body burden in humans. This decision precipitated including, for the first time in any recognized toxicology text, a chapter on the predicted intake of mercury vapor from amalgam dental fillings. The chapter is included in the text book *The Biological Monitoring of Toxic Metals* (3) and makes the following six conclusions about the release of mercury from amalgam fillings:

1. The evidence indicates that amalgam surfaces release mercury vapor into the mouth.

2. The rate of release is increased by stressing the amalgam surface by chewing and brushing.

3. The surface layer does not immediately repair after stress and that it may take several hours to completely restore the surface layer. [Bio-Probe NOTE: The authors are saying that once the filling is stimulated by chewing, brushing, etc., it starts releasing increased amounts of mercury vapor and that it may take several hours before the release rate is reduced back to the static or unstimulated value.]

4. The release of mercury from amalgam results in the deposition of mercury in body tissue and an increase in urinary excretion.

5. The estimated release rates from amalgam appear to be consistent with levels of mercury found in autopsy tissue in the general population and with increases in brain and urinary levels due to amalgam fillings.

6. The release of mercury from dental amalgams makes the predominant contribution to human exposure to inorganic mercury including mercury vapor in the general population.

Confirmation of the above conclusions are contained in the recently published World Health Organization (WHO) Environmental Health Criteria 118 document titled "Inorganic Mercury."(4) Table 2 on page 36 of the 118 criteria document displays the following information:

Table 2. Estimated average daily intake and retention (ug/day) of total mercury and mercury compounds in the general population not occupationally exposed to mercury[a]

Exposure	Elemental mercury vapour	Inorganic mercury compounds	Methylmercury
Air	0.030 (0.024)	0.002 (0.001)	0.008 (0.0064)
Food			
Fish	0	0.600 (0.042)	2.4 (2.3)
Non-fish	0	3.6 (0.25)	0
Drinking-water	0	0.050 (0.0035)	0
Dental amalgams	3.8-21 (3-17)	0	0
Total	3.9-21 (3.1-17)	4.3 (0.3)	2.41 (2.31)

[a] From: Environmental Health Criteria 101: Methylmercury (WHO 1990)

Values given are the estimated average daily intake; the figures in parentheses represent the estimated amount retained in the body of an adult.

Values are quoted to 2 significant figures.

There is an important phenomenon that has not received the proper degree of attention. It occurs when gold and amalgam are present together in the mouth When these two metals are present at the same time in the oral cavity the resulting electric currents that are generated cause an increased release of mercury from the amalgam regardless of whether or not the amalgam is visible. Often amalgam cores are used under gold crowns or gold bridges are placed directly on amalgam filled teeth. A dark discoloration of the tooth and adjacent gum tissue is sometimes visible, indicating migration of amalgam components. If the amalgam filling is in direct contact with gold, it can sometimes evaporate more mercury than all other amalgam fillings together. When gold is placed on top of amalgam, mercury will migrate and the tissues surrounding the tooth can have extremely high levels of mercury. (5,6)

If you have silver/mercury dental fillings your biochemical individuality, diet and lifestyle assume much greater importance. These factors provide the rationale of why some people with amalgam fillings cope with the extra daily intake of mercury vapor and why some people do not. It is in the "do not" group where signs and symptoms of mercury toxicity, resulting from an inability to cope with the additional chronic intake of mercury vapor from dental fillings, begins to appear. In other words, their bodies are no longer capable of biochemically detoxifying the added burden of mercury.

The natural question that follows is: What can I do about it? or: What can I do to help reduce or minimize the effects of chronic exposure to mercury vapor? If you were asking those questions of a toxicologist, the first course of action recommended would be to eliminate the source of exposure and the second course of action would be to therapeutically attempt to reduce the body burden of mercury.

In the situation we are addressing, the source of mercury that would have to be eliminated is the silver/mercury dental fillings. However, and unfortunately for many people, this becomes a purely financial decision. Consequently, for many people their immediate concern centers around the question: Is there anything I can do now to help myself without having my amalgams replaced?

The answer to that question is a qualified yes. Qualified because no matter what program is instituted to overcome the destructive metabolic effects of mercury, it is irrational to assume that the source does not have to be eliminated even though there is some relief or improvement in health. The average adult human takes at least 17,000 breaths of air per day. If you have silver/mercury dental fillings, this means that you are inhaling 17,000 micro-doses of mercury vapor each day. It takes the body about 30-70 days to get rid of 1/2 of a single dose of mercury vapor exposure. This means that as long as you have a source of mercury vapor implanted in your teeth your body will continue to very slowly accumulate mercury, adding to your total body burden of this insidious poison.(7)

Therapeutically, there are different approaches available. For example, there are drugs on the market that have a

8

great affinity for mercury and will help reduce body burdens. The same can also be said for different homeopathic remedies. Both of these, however, have to be administered under the supervision of a physician or licensed health professional. Nutrition is the only therapeutic option easily available for self-help.

SUPPLEMENTS

Do not expect supplements to act like medicines, which rapidly take away the symptoms without doing anything to the underlying cause. Supplements are intended to correct deficiencies and to enhance your resistance to harmful influences. If you are healthy, not exposed to toxic compounds and eat a varied diet, you have no immediate need for supplements but your performance is likely to be enhanced by moderate doses. Unfortunately, everyone is exposed to metals, other toxic substances and stress. The ideal situation does not really exist. Everyone has a unique metabolism and might need more of a particular supplement. Modern farming, food manufacturing, and cooking changes the food, leading to oxidation and loss of vitamins and trace elements. In processed foods some of these, but not all, are added again. Recommended intakes of vitamins are based on levels which prevent deficiency diseases, not on intakes which should give optimum health. If there also is a load of toxic substances, your body will utilize more of the protective substances and more will be needed each day. Requirements are conditional, depending on what you are exposed to, your lifestyle, genetic factors etc. Even for a professional nutritionist it will be very difficult, or directly impossible to figure out what to eat to get optimum intakes of every vitamin and mineral.

At the present time, the most comprehensive single source of scientific information detailing how mercury can disrupt biochemical pathways and cause nutritional deficiencies is contained in Chapter 11 of the book *Infertility & Birth Defects - Is Mercury From Silver Dental Fillings an Unsuspected Cause?*(8)

Attempting to reverse the process, by supplementing with those nutrients being affected the most by mercury, appears to be one way of reducing some of the effects of chronic exposure. Many of the nutrients also have an ability to bind with mercury and lead, which would then tend to help your body excrete these toxic metals, thereby reducing your total body burden. (Reference to lead has been included because it is universally available in the air we breath and in our food chain and affects many of the same biochemical pathways as mercury.)

There are several nutrient manufacturers in this country that have recognized the necessity of providing products that will assist in reducing body burdens of heavy metals and/or environmental pollutants. Most health food stores throughout the country carry some of these products, and store personnel are usually able to advise you of the manufacturers' technical information evolved from testing or the scientific literature related to formulation of the product.

There are some other aspects of nutritional supplementation that can be of great significance in the efficacy of their use.

The first deals with whether the particular brand you bought has been manufactured and tested to insure that the tablet dissolves after you have swallowed it. For a nutritional supplement to be of any use to you it should dissolve in about thirty minutes. Unfortunately, many supplements are made so hard and insoluble that they may pass through the entire gastrointestinal tract without ever beginning to dissolve. Consequently, such tablets will be of little benefit in any detoxification program.

If you suspect that your supplements are not dissolving properly, inquire at the store where you purchased the items, asking them to provide you with information regarding the standards of disintegration used by the manufacturer. If you are unable to obtain this information from the store where you purchased the supplements, you can call the manufacturer yourself. Or, there is a simple home test you can do yourself that will give you a fairly accurate evaluation as to whether or not your supplements are dissolving. Place your tablet in a glass of lukewarm water to which a little vinegar has been added. Without touching the tablet, stir the water at short intervals. The tablet should dissolve in less than one hour. If it doesn't dissolve within an hour it means that it will be of little nutritional benefit to you and in fact may cause some problems by remaining in the lower intestines, where it can putrefy or irritate the digestive tract.

Another major problem deals with when you take supplements. Some people take their supplements on an empty stomach, others take them before meals, or after meals, etc. By definition, the word supplement means to "supply a deficiency." Therefore our basic concern is how to get the most benefit from a supplement in correcting a deficiency. The assimilation of some nutrients is facilitated by taking them before your meal, so that the full effect of your stomach acids can start the digestion process without being diluted by food. Others are fat soluble vitamins, which means that they require some fat and fat digesting enzymes in order for the body to handle them properly. Fat soluble nutrients are best taken after a meal. Still others, such as amino acids and acidophilus, are best taken on an empty stomach so they do not have to compete with amino acids in foods or have the food detract from their full effect. Throughout the balance of this book, where we refer to the supplements you should take we have included available information indicating the most effective time for consumption.

The information on supplements contained in this book is not intended as medical advice. Rather, it is an interpretation of some of the scientific information contained in Chapter 11 of *Infertility & Birth Defects,* the *Bio-Probe Newsletter*, and other pertinent scientific literature. Ideally, your effort to improve your nutritional status should be under the direction of a qualified physician or health care professional. This is especially true for those individuals who are presently allergic to a variety of substances. Individuals electing to self-experiment should do so with caution.

As a general caution with regard to embarking on a nutritional supplementation program--don't be in a hurry. The body has a very delicate balance mechanism and unless you are well read on nutrition and are presently supplementing, proceed slowly, giving your body a chance to adjust as you add new nutrients.

SELF-EVALUATION PROGRAM

In some people the addition of some of the key nutrients affected by mercury and lead may produce some beneficial health effects through the reduction of some symptomatology related to existing health problems. Although this does not constitute scientific proof that mercury from your mercury/silver dental fillings is the culprit, it does suggest that you may be on the right track. The following represents a simple program that you may wish to initially try for a period of four to six weeks. If you feel better and have an abatement of symptoms, it may be indicative of a possible correlation to your silver/mercury dental fillings.

SPECIAL NOTE: Those individuals with occlusal mercury/silver fillings should stop chewing gum. The chewing forces involved will continually stimulate the release of mercury vapor from the fillings, adding substantially to your body burden of mercury.

Mercury will attach to sulfur amino acid building blocks in proteins. The sulfur amino acids are methionine, cysteine, and taurine. There is also a sulfur-containing tripeptide (having three amino acids) called glutathione that is composed of glutamic acid, cysteine, and glycine. Sulfur is present in all proteins. Numerous enzymes require intact sulfur groups and many are inactivated by mercury. Cysteine reacts readily with many substances and recent research indicates that there may be some problems with supplementing with cysteine. Therefore, we are now recommending that cysteine supplements not be taken until further scientific research clarifies the situation. Until that

12

time, we suggest that you use methionine and glutathione as primary sulfur sources. Your body can produce cysteine from methionine and glutathione provides cysteine in a form that is less reactive.

1. Glutathione (GSH). The reason for starting with glutathione is that when any type of detoxification activity is undertaken, there is usually a tissue redistribution of heavy metals within the body. This can result in additional mercury being taken up by the brain, which could aggravate some of your symptoms. If you have actually been experiencing toxic effects of mercury, your available supply of glutathione would also be reduced. In this regard, a recent book on amino acids states "GSH also protects against mercury toxicity. At the age of two to four weeks, the body becomes capable of excreting mercury through the bile. This correlates with the increasing ability of the liver to secrete glutathione. It is no accident that GSH deficiency resulting from genetic errors mimics the acute mercury toxicity effects of Minamata disease. Without adequate GSH, mercury from the environment cannot be detoxified and eliminated."(9) [Bio-Probe NOTE: The authors were evidently unaware of the significant contribution to mercury body burden made by amalgam dental fillings. However, the last sentence of the quotation demonstrates the critical necessity of having an adequate supply of glutathione to be able to detoxify the additional chemical insult being caused by the release of mercury from amalgams.]

Therefore, the first nutrient you should supplement is glutathione, which will help replenish your supply and should also minimize any effects related to redistribution. It usually comes in a 50 milligram tablet or capsule and you should start taking 50 milligrams three times a day on an empty stomach. (Amino acids are best taken on an empty stomach to avoid competing with those contained in your food.) You can take it between meals, before going to bed, or upon awakening in the morning. Take only glutathione for the first 3-4 days before you add the next nutrient.

13

2. N-Acetyl-L-Cysteine (NAC). NAC forms L-cysteine, cystine, L-methionine, glutathione (GSH), and mixed di-sulfides. This compound (used by the medical profession to treat acetaminophen overdose) has the ability of being able to stimulate your own body to produce large amounts of cysteine and glutathione, thus greatly augmenting plasma and red blood cell content of both cysteine and glutathione.(10) In experiments where animals were exposed to mercury vapor, NAC treatment increased survival time and decreased mercury levels in blood, lung and kidney. (11,12) Therefore, you may wish to try NAC to augment your body's ability to produce additional cysteine and glutathione. As with the other nutrients, you should try NAC three or four days after starting glutathione to insure you do not have any type of reaction to it.

3. Methylsulfonylmethane (MSM)® is a natural dietary sulfur compound that provides bioavailable sulfur. This product can provide sulfur to cysteine and methionine. MSM is a natural form of organic sulfur found in all living organisms and is completely free of odor or after-taste. Mercury's great affinity for the sulfur molecule makes MSM a valuable, readily available, source of dietary sulfur. Sulfur labeled MSM has been found to be incorporated into protein cysteine residues throughout the body.(13) MSM should therefore be a valuable adjunct in helping to offset the toxic effects of chronic mercury exposure.

MSM® is the registered trademark for licensed methylsulfonylmethane U.S. Patent No. 4,616,039. It is being provided as a nutritional supplement by Advanced Medical Nutrition, Inc. (AMNI). Their toll-free number is 1-800-356-4791

4. Vitamin B_6 (Pyridoxine). Three or four days after starting glutathione supplementation (and NAC if you elect to try it), your next nutrient should be Vitamin B_6. Vitamin B_6 is critically involved in the metabolism of the sulfur amino acids. This is especially true in the conversion of one amino acid to another. For example, B_6 is needed in the metabolic processes that convert methionine to cysteine

14

to glutathione. Therefore, having an adequate intake of vitamin B_6 will help insure that your body has the needed nutrients to produce cysteine and convert it to additional glutathione. It is suggested you take one 50 mg B_6 tablet per day with your breakfast meal. NOTE: There have been a few published cases of high doses of vitamin B_6 producing reversible disturbances of the peripheral nervous system. Chronic high dose usage should only be done under your physicians supervision.

5. Zinc is the next nutrient to be added. Zinc stimulates the production of metallothionein in the body, which is one way the body detoxifies the effects of mercury. (Metallothionein is very rich in cysteine). There are several different kinds of zinc available, all with different potencies. It is suggested that you take one zinc tablet per day with a meal and the potency can be 15-30 milligrams. After you have been taking the glutathione and vitamin B_6 for 3-4 days, add the one zinc tablet per day to your regimen. Continue the three items for an additional 3-4 days, closely observing for any changes.

6. Vitamin C is the next nutrient to be added. Prolonged exposures to low mercury concentrations tend to depress the adrenal ascorbic acid content. Providing additional vitamin C should help restore and/or maintain adequate adrenal levels of this critical nutrient, thus tending to offset the depletion by chemical stress caused by chronic inhalation of mercury vapor. There are many forms of vitamin C, from plain ascorbic acid to those buffered with calcium or magnesium. There are also various types of hypoallergenic vitamin C made from different raw materials. Whichever product you select, start out with 500 milligrams per day, taken with a meal. After 3-4 days, start increasing your dosage until you are taking 1500 milligrams per day in divided doses.

7. Vitamin B_1 (thiamine) is the next nutrient to be added, 3-4 days after vitamin C. Use a 50-milligram tablet and take one tablet with each meal for a total of 150 milligrams per day.

B-vitamins are involved in energy metabolism, supporting the systems which protect against free radicals. Vitamin B_1 also contains a sulfur group and has been used (50-100 mg intramuscular injection) to treat mercury poisoning. The vitamin has a rapid turnover in the brain and the levels are reduced by mercury exposure (mercury oxidizes thiamine to thiochrome).(14) The symptoms of B_1 deficiency and mercury poisoning are almost identical.

8. Selenium is the last nutrient to be added. Selenium binds with mercury and will start to cause a redistribution of tissue mercury. It should also precipitate some excretion of mercury from the body. Selenium is available in several forms and potencies. Inorganic selenium is the substance which has been used to protect experimental animals from mercury poisoning. If you take inorganic selenium you will not risk a slow build-up of tissue selenium, since excess is excreted in urine. Organic selenium, on the other hand, is incorporated into a variety of proteins instead of the sulfur-containing methionine. Proteins have a turnover of some months and it is therefore possible to build up a store of selenium. It is suggested that you start with a 50-microgram tablet three times a day for a total of 150 micrograms daily. PLEASE NOTE: Selenium should not be taken with vitamin C. Take your selenium between meals or whenever possible, two hours before or after you have taken vitamin C.

For those who are allergic to yeast derived products, sodium selenite in tablet or liquid form is available. (Liquid selenium is available from Nutricolgy, Inc. (Allergy Research Group) 1-800-545-9960 Ext. 200. Individuals who are sensitive to petrochemicals sometimes react to small quantities of selenium and should either be under the guidance of a physician or initiate selenium supplementation very slowly. Those individuals who react to selenium may experience dizziness or an upset stomach. However, if they are not allergic to selenium these types of reactions should clear in a few days. Do not take more than 50 micrograms per day until you have established that you are experiencing no adverse allergic reaction.

Some people may have beneficial health effects, from the indicated supplementation, within the first week; in others, it may take 60-90 days to notice any improvement. There is also the chance that you won't experience any benefit. However, it is a non-invasive, cost effective way to do a little health-detective work. Improvements in sense of well-being, energy levels, and amelioration of any existing symptomatology are all positive indications that your nutriture of glutathione, pyridoxine, zinc, vitamin C, thiamine and selenium had been impaired. This does not mean, categorically, that mercury and/or lead were the cause. However, it does indicate that serious consideration should be given to that possibility.

DIETARY CHANGES

Assuming you have achieved some beneficial effects from your supplementation program, what else can you do to help your body cope more effectively with the stress of heavy metal exposure?

First, and foremost, is the consideration of dietary changes that might help in the overall goal of reducing intake and increasing excretion. The largest dietary source of mercury comes from fish and fish products. You should become very selective about the amount and type of fish you eat. Limited data available indicates that some fish have comparatively lower mercury contents. Some of these are sardines, herring, pollack, mackerel, cod, redfish, and Greenland halibut. Most tuna has a fairly high content of mercury and, even though selenium levels in tuna may offset the effects of the mercury, discretion dictates avoiding tuna during any mercury detoxification program. Intake of shellfish should also be eliminated or greatly reduced as shellfish are scavengers and usually contain high levels of heavy metals. Patient case histories indicate that individuals who are sensitive to mercury usually have some type of adverse reaction from shellfish.

There is another aspect related to fish products that mercury sensitive individuals must consider. Fish meal has become a major feed for chickens. Consequently,

17

depending on the mercury content of the fish products used to make the fish meal, chickens and eggs have the potential of having a significant mercury content. We have patient reports indicating that chicken and eggs can exacerbate symptoms in individuals with known sensitivities to mercury.

You can also ensure that you routinely eat a high-fiber diet. This will tend to decrease fecal transit time, reducing the amount of time that liquids containing heavy metals remain in the colon. This will reduce the quantity reabsorbed from the colon, which passes through the portal vein into the liver and is then recirculated throughout the body. SPECIAL NOTE: High fiber diets may contain excessive amounts of phytic acid which binds zinc and can lead to a zinc deficiency.(15) You should have a physician check your zinc levels as you may require extra zinc to maintain a proper zinc ratio. (See Appendix A for a simple home zinc status test). A study by Rowland et al. in 1986 demonstrated the significance of fiber. Utilizing mice that had been exposed to methylmercury, the study set out to determine if fiber made any difference in the whole-body retention of mercury. The incorporation of 30% wheat bran in the diet of the mice significantly decreased the total mercury concentration in the brain, blood, and small intestine. The authors felt that wheat bran exerted its effects on mercury retention and brain level via a modification of the metabolic activity of the gut microflora.(16) Recent research by Dr. A. Summers and her associates at the University of Georgia has established that bacteria in the gut of animals with amalgam fillings can become "mercury resistant." The significance of this is that these bacteria can convert various forms of mercury into mercury vapor which can then be reabsorbed and recirculated in the blood to the brain and other critical organs in the body. This can also lead to antibiotic resistance, which is becoming a very serious problem to the medical profession.(17) It appears that a high fiber diet will cause the excretion of large quantities of mercury resistant bacteria in the feces, thus reducing the amount of mercury vapor to be recirculated.

Although there has not been any specific research with oat bran and mercury that we are aware of, oat bran added to the diet may be equally as beneficial because of the cysteine and methionine content. Oat bran also provides the added benefit of reducing cholesterol levels. Researchers feel that oat bran increases the excretion of bile acids, which are made from cholesterol, as well as increasing the excretion of bile in the feces.(18) As mercury is carried by the bile into the intestine, an adequate fiber intake decreases the amount of mercury available to be recycled back to the liver. A simple way to get additional fiber is to eat oat or bran muffins. For anyone taking supplementary fiber it is important that an adequate amount of water be consumed and that you build up the amount of fiber consumed very slowly. Taking excessive fiber can have the opposite effect and result in serious blockage in the large colon. Additionally, routine intakes of 6-8 glasses of non-fluoridated water daily will also assist your body in getting rid of toxins.

The status of your intestinal flora also plays a significant role in the excretion of both methylmercury and inorganic mercury in your feces. Stress and use of antibiotics can reduce viable strains of intestinal bacteria and cause overgrowth of undesirable strains, in essence reducing the quality of the intestinal flora. One way the body rids itself of mercury is via the bile which empties into your intestine. If your intestinal flora is impaired, then mercury, and for that matter other heavy metals that would have been excreted in your feces, are recirculated back to the liver. Including items in your diet that are rich in favorable bacteria, such as unsweetened yogurt with live cultures, acidophilus supplements, buttermilk and other soured milk products, will assist in the maintenance of your intestinal flora.

For a further discussion of a high fibre diet protocol to cleanse the colon of heavy metals see Appendix B.

DIETARY SOURCES OF PARTICULAR NUTRIENTS

Foods are listed in decreasing order of content:

1. Selenium: Butter, smoked herring, Brazil nuts, cashew nuts, wheat germ and bran, scallops, barley, whole wheat bread, milk, brown rice, brewers yeast, oats, garlic, cheddar cheese, and molasses.

2. Zinc: Herring, sunflower seeds, pumpkin seeds, ground round steak, lamb chops, pecans, Brazil nuts, beef liver, egg yolk, whole wheat bread, oats, almonds, sardines, and chicken.

3. Thiamine: Wheat germ, rice bran, yeast, ham, dried raisins and prunes, asparagus, beans, broccoli, cauliflower, corn, lentils, brown rice, almonds, cashews, and eggs.

4. Methionine and Cysteine: NOTE: The determination of sulfur-amino acid content of various foods is not readily available. As a general rule, recommendations as good food sources of sulfur-containing amino acids have been wheat germ, yogurt, cottage cheese, pork, sausage meat, turkey, eggs, beans, brussels sprouts, onions, garlic, hot red peppers, horseradish,cabbage, brown rice, sesame seeds, pumpkin seeds, oat flakes, granola and avocado.

Dietary intake of refined carbohydrates, sugars, and saturated fats should be reduced. These types of foods have high energy requirements for metabolism and may well reduce the availability of essential enzymes and nutrients required for more beneficial purposes.

PHARMACEUTICALS

You should also become very critical of every pharmaceutical product you use, prescription or over-the-counter, with regard to whether it contains mercury in any form. The same can be said for cosmetic products, many of which still contain some forms of mercury. In the past, a great many ophthalmic solutions contained thimerosal (which contains mercury) as an antibacterial agent. However, a recent check of solutions for contact lenses revealed that the number containing mercury had been greatly reduced. Substitutes should be used for merthiolate or mercurochrome. In this regard, patients who are undergoing periodic or a series of injections of nutrients and/or drugs, under your physicians direction, should insure that the multi-dose vial of the injectable does not contain thimerosal as a preservative. All multi-dose injectables contain some preservative and the use of thimerosal is very common. There are several over-the-counter ointments as well as some ophthalmic ointments or eye salves that contain yellow mercuric oxide or ammoniated mercury. There are also other ointments that contain calomel (mercurous chloride). Some cathartic pills also contain calomel. You will find antiseptic creams or lotions that contain ammoniated mercury. Many skin bleaching preparations contain ammoniated mercury. Some long acting nasal sprays may contain mercury in the form of thimerosal (merthiolate). As you can see from the range of products, it is important that you start reading labels and asking questions. Be observant of ingredients on labels; the letters "-mer-" in various combinations usually means mercury.

LIFESTYLE CHANGES

Within this category there are many things that can be done that will augment any effects being achieved through nutritional supplementation and diet modification. Perhaps the most important is to make every effort to reduce the degree or amount of stress to which your body is routinely subjected. This is essential because stress depletes your body of key nutrients.

If you are not exercising then you should establish some schedule for yourself that results in you performing some type of physical exercise at least three times a week, with each session being at least thirty minutes in duration. However, be very cautious in initiating any exercise regimen, particularly if you have any physical or health problem. Moreover, if your body's normal metabolic performance has been weakened, as it might be from mercury accumulation, the additional stress derived from exercise may be detrimental. Be certain to consult with and obtain approval from your physician before initiating any exercise program.

Aside from the physiological benefits of exercise in this instance, there is a more immediate detoxifying benefit that will accrue if you "work up a sweat". Sweat is one of the body's mechanisms for getting rid of toxins, including some heavy metals like mercury. In fact, induced sweating is the therapeutic modality used to detoxify workers employed at the mercury mines in Spain who have suffered excessive exposure. Sweating can also be induced by taking periodic steam baths or saunas, providing your doctor approves. There has been some anecdotal evidence that some individuals react to steam/sauna induced sweating, getting flu like symptoms or other mercury toxic symptoms. There has also been one case of Exercise Induced Anaphylaxis (EIA) reported in the literature, which improved after removal of amalgam fillings.(19) EIA warning symptoms are: generalized body warmth, itching, and erythema (redness of the skin) that progresses on continued exertion to confluent urticaria, angioedema, gastrointestinal symptoms, headache and sometimes unconsciousness. Bio-Probe NOTE: We feel that in both types of induced sweating, individuals are re-inhaling mercury vapor coming off of the mercury being eliminated in the perspiration. There could also be some type of systemic reaction occurring at the same time. Anytime your body starts dumping mercury there is a cellular redistribution that occurs. Mercury will be coming out of the cells into the blood, where some will be excreted and some will be redeposited at new sites in the body, causing either an allergic reaction or some other systemic reaction.

Giving up smoking and the consumption of alcoholic beverages would also assist and augment your other efforts. However, that is easier said than done for most people. Conversely, most people can, without too much trouble or inconvenience, reduce their intake or use of tobacco and alcohol without causing any particular mental stress. It appears that the benefit from limiting or stopping is associated with reducing the chemical stress on the body, which biochemically uses many of the same nutrients you are trying to use to rid or reduce your burden of mercury.

REPLACEMENT PROTOCOLS

WHAT TO DO IF PRESENTLY PREGNANT

If you are presently pregnant, the most important question to arise will be: What should I do about dental work or the replacement of mercury amalgam dental fillings? This is also the most difficult decision confronting your dentist or physician. There is no scientific evidence that provides a definitive answer to the question. Consequently, there are differing views.

One view is that mercury amalgam fillings should not be replaced during pregnancy because of the potential temporary increased mercury body burden that might result. This might increase the potential of toxic effects occurring to the embryo or fetus, particularly if it occurs during the first trimester of pregnancy. Therefore, as has been stated by some of the world leaders on mercury toxicology, comprehensive amalgam work on pregnant women should not be performed. In effect, only dental care deemed absolutely essential should be provided, and amalgam is not to be used for any of the work that must be done.

The differing view is that elimination of the mercury source at the outset of pregnancy is the lesser of two evils. This view holds that the continuous release and inhalation of mercury from mercury amalgam dental fillings for the entire term of the pregnancy and nursing can present a greater hazard to the mother, fetus, and child, than would the amount of exposure resulting from replacement. A recent animal study by Dr. M. J. Vimy and his associates at the University of Calgary School of Medicine in Canada has shown that breast milk concentrates mercury and contains up to six times more mercury than that in the mother's blood.(20)

As you can see, it is not an easy decision, nor one that can be taken lightly. Sadly, there is no scientific data upon which to make a decision. No studies have ever been done to determine what the potential body burdens of mercury are that would accrue from replacement done at the beginning of pregnancy compared to calculations of total mercury accrual during the nine months of pregnancy and approximately nine months of nursing.

There is, however, some scientific data that weighs heavily on the decision process. These relate to the critical periods of development during the reproductive cycle. It would appear from the data available that any additional unnecessary mercury exposure during these critical periods of embryonic or fetal growth could have devastating results.

Consequently, we share the position taken by the Swedish Expert Commission and the World Health Organization that mercury exposure during pregnancy should be avoided. Within that frame of reference, and until scientific research is available to the contrary, we believe that dental work during pregnancy should be confined to only that which is absolutely essential. Unless considered absolutely necessary by your physician and dentist, all dental work should be avoided during the first trimester. Another animal study at the University of Calgary School of Medicine by L.J. Hahn and associates has clearly demonstrated accumulation of mercury in the fetus within two days of having amalgam fillings placed.(20)

Having taken that position does not mean that there is nothing further to be done about the mercury problem. Quite the contrary, every effort should be made to reduce or control your mercury body burden during pregnancy. As discussed previously, stop chewing gum, eat a diet rich in sulfur-containing foods, discuss with your physician which supplements you can take and in what quantities, and finally, limit your intake of fish and seafood. With regard to the amount of mercury that can be passed to the child through breast feeding, it should be noted that selenium supplements have been shown to decrease the mercury content of breast milk.(21)

WHAT TO DO IF PLANNING A FAMILY

What actions should be taken if you are planning a pregnancy? Here we feel the decision is much simpler, assuming that you have made the decision to have your mercury amalgam dental fillings replaced. Based on the scientific data available, we would recommend that amalgam replacement for both the husband and wife should be completed six months prior to attempting conception. The six-month period following final amalgam replacement will permit your body burden of mercury to reduce and your body chemistry to re-balance or adjust. Another important aspect of improving the balance of nutrients relates to recent animal studies demonstrating that parental zinc and selenium deficiencies prior to conception have an adverse effect on the immune system of the offspring.(22,23)

SUPPLEMENTATION DURING AND AFTER AMALGAM REPLACEMENT

A question we are frequently asked concerns supplementation programs prior to, as well as after amalgam replacement. To help your body in detoxifying or reducing any existing body burden of mercury and to also assist you in coping with any additional exposure that might result from amalgam removal, the following regimen provides the nutrients that, based on the scientific literature, may be of help. This should not be confused with the program previously outlined which was designed to determine if mercury was involved in the etiology of any symptoms you might have had.

PRE-AMALGAM REPLACEMENT

Should be started as soon as possible but no later than two weeks prior to first amalgam replacement.

1. Glutathione: One 50 milligram capsule or tablet, three times a day taken on an empty stomach.

2. Methionine: One 200-500 milligram tablet three times a day on the same schedule indicated for glutathione. As with all new supplements added to your program, it is prudent to start out taking only one tablet a day for the first three or four days to insure that you are not having any reaction. If no problems are experienced then add the second and third tablets. The importance of adding methionine to your detoxification program is explained nicely by Dr's. Braverman and Pfeiffer in the following statement: "Glutathione contains cysteine, glycine and glutamic acid, but of these, only cysteine ever seems to be in short supply...The liver apparently manufactures glutathione whenever extra cysteine is available. Blood glutathione levels change in direct proportion to the amount of cysteine in the diet."(9) As methionine is the precursor for the manufacture of cysteine in the body, extra supplementation of this critical amino acid should increase available cysteine.

3. N-Acetyl-L-Cysteine (NAC). NAC forms L-cysteine, cystine, L-methionine, glutathione (GSH), and mixed di-sulfides. This compound (used by the medical profession to treat acetaminophen overdose) has the ability of being able to stimulate your own body to produce large amounts of cysteine and glutathione, thus greatly augmenting plasma and red blood cell content of both cysteine and glutathione.(10) In experiments where animals were exposed to mercury vapor, NAC treatment increased survival time and decreased mercury levels in blood, lung and kidney. (11,12)

4. Methylsulfonylmethane MSM®. We have added this product because it provides a bioavailable dietary source of sulfur. MSM which contains other ingredients besides sulfur, can exert a direct beneficial effect in ameliorating a variety of allergic responses and pain associated with systemic inflammatory disorders.(13) Although at this time we have no published research outlining its use in mercury

toxicity, there is a wealth of data demonstrating the essentialness of sulfur in the formation of disulfide bonds and the proper conformation of body proteins. This in turn provides the biochemical basis for its inclusion in this protocol. Another very important rationale for its inclusion in our detoxification protocol is that Frederik Berglund, M.D. in Sweden has been using elemental sulfur in treating amalgam bearers after exchange of their mercury-containing fillings. It is our understanding that positive results are being achieved especially for problems associated with gastrointestinal functions and the eyes. It is possible that as more experience is obtained in the use of MSM® in the treatment of mercury toxicity, it may assume a primary role in mercury detoxification. The recommended maintenance dose of MSM is 500-2000 mg per day.

5. Vitamin B_6 (Pyridoxine): One 50 milligram tablet per day with breakfast. B_6 is needed in the metabolic process that convert methionine to cysteine and then into glutathione. NOTE: Clinical experience has demonstrated that vitamin B6 is capable of reducing and controlling the swelling and pain associated with the routine tissue and bone trauma resulting from normal dental operative procedures. Typical dosages used to assist in the reduction of post-operative swelling have been 100 to 200 milligrams one hour prior to dental work, and an additional 100 to 200 milligrams after you get home from the dental office. This can be followed the next day with 200-300 milligrams more if the swelling has persisted.

Do not use the dosages indicated for more than 3-4 days. Supplementation at high doses for any prolonged period should only be done under your physician's supervision.

6. Vitamin C: One 500 milligram tablet with each meal. It should be noted that most vitamin C products are derived from corn. If you have known allergies to corn, there are products available made out of Sago Palm. [NOTE: Clinical experience has shown that in some individuals, vitamin C can affect the way they respond to dental anesthesia. In

some, the anesthetizing effects are dissipated more quickly than desired, while in others the dentist is unable to anesthetize the work area at all. Therefore, as a general guideline, do not take any vitamin C for 12 hours before your scheduled dental appointment.]

7. Zinc: One 15-30 milligram tablet after supper.

8. Magnesium: One tablet per day providing 100 milligrams of elemental magnesium, taken after supper or at bed time. Please read the label. Labels on minerals will usually state the total number of milligrams of the mineral it takes to provide the elemental dosage.

9. Vitamin B_1: One 50 milligram tablet with each meal.

On the day of your dental appointment you may wish to increase your dosage of vitamin B1 to 200-500 milligrams one hour before your dental appointment. Research has shown that vitamin B1 is capable of reducing pain that may be associated with routine dental operative procedures.(24) Increased dosages may be used the following day to assist in controlling residual pain. Although we have not seen any research specifically applied to the use of vitamin B1 for reduction of mercury body burden, there is a study demonstrating that 2000 milligrams per day was very effective in reducing the body burden of lead. Lead, as you know, has many of the same biochemical pathways as mercury.(25) As with any supplement or medication, do not stay on high intakes for any extended period without consultation with your physician.

10. Add Vitamin E. If you have previously taken vitamin E and experienced no blood pressure changes, then you can supplement with 100-400 IU capsules. The desired dosage should be 800-1200 IU per day. If you have previously experienced any adverse blood pressure reaction with vitamin E, then you should start with the lowest potency available and take no more than 50-100 IU per day for the first 30 days. Discontinue taking vitamin E if at any time you experience an adverse reaction or increase in blood pressure. For those individuals who are very

allergic, care should be exercised with regard to the derivative source of the vitamin E; for example, the soya bean is a common source of vitamin E because of the availability of the raw material, wheat is the next most important source, etc. Insure that you get a product to which you are not allergic to. Products of oxidation such as lipid peroxides, which can be caused by mercury, are converted to harmless products by vitamin E and glutathione peroxidase (a selenium containing enzyme derived from glutathione and selenium). Wheat germ oil, sunflower seeds, safflower oil, almonds, sesame oil, peanut oil, corn oil, wheat germ, peanuts, olive oil, soybean oil and peanut butter are food sources of vitamin E in descending order of highest occurrence.(26)

11. Selenium: One 50 microgram tablet (or liquid equivalent of sodium selenite). Vitamin C precipitates selenium, making it unavailable for absorption. The two supplements should be taken at least two hours apart from each other. As stated earlier, some individuals may react adversely to selenium, so caution should be exercised. (Note: Some manufacturers now provide products combining both selenium and vitamin E).

12. Acidophilus capsules, powder, or liquid: Acidophilus, or yogurt with live acidophilus culture, taken regularly will help restore the microflora of the intestine which can be adversely affected by the presence of mercury in any form. Aside from the mercury related aspects, acidophilus has been shown to: "reduce bad breath by replacing organisms responsible for unpleasant odors with neutral organisms; reduce flatulence (intestinal gas) by breaking down sugars (including lactose) that promote and are consumed by methane-producing bacteria; regulate cholesterol by promoting normal absorption of dietary fats, facilitate the elimination of unwanted cholesterol before its absorbed;and provide adaptogenic control (normalization) of constipation and diarrhea."(27) Please read the product information to determine when you should take the particular supplement you are purchasing.

The above comprises the primary nutrients that have been scientifically shown to assist in the elimination of mercury from the body or to afford some degree of protection from mercury induced damage. In addition, the following products have all been shown to be of benefit and their addition to any program is at the reader's option:

13. B Complex: Should provide at least 15-25 milligrams of each of the various B vitamins. Take the number of tablets indicated to provide the desired amounts. [NOTE: A word of caution concerning those individuals taking large amounts or injections of vitamin B_{12}. There is limited scientific information indicating that vitamin B_{12} can methylate mercury. Consequently, during the entire amalgam replacement process, every effort should be made to eliminate excess B_{12} intake. If you must receive B_{12} injections, request your physician to use hydroxocobalamin.]

14. Activated charcoal, taken immediately before drilling/chunking out amalgam, will bind any swallowed mercury and also prevent enterohepatic recirculation of the metal (excretion with the bile and reabsorption further down the intestines). There is some evidence that NAC and methionine will adsorb to charcoal, reducing their availability. Therefore, charcoal should not be routinely used in your detoxification program other than during dental appointments, where the increased potential of mercury exposure exists.

15. Garlic products contain high levels of sulfur and some contain selenium. Research has shown that garlic protects against many harmful conditions including mercury poisoning. Most preparations on the market today are odor free.

16. Bromelain: Bromelain is a powerful proteolytic enzyme derived from pineapple. Clinical evidence indicates it can help reduce swelling and inflammation.(28) If you are going to use it to help minimize any swelling or inflammation that may result from dental operative procedures, a couple of days before your dental

30

appointment take 500 mg of bromelain twice daily. Take between meals with a full glass of water.

SPECIAL NOTE: As indicated earlier under the supplementation section, the ideal situation is to be under the care and supervision of a qualified physician or health professional. In this regard, unless your physician has specifically prescribed iron and copper supplements for you, please refrain from taking any supplement that contains iron and copper. If you are starting on your own program and have not been taking vitamin supplements, it is important that you phase slowly into the program, giving your body a chance to adjust and balance to the changes.

POST-AMALGAM REPLACEMENT

If, after amalgam replacement, you are not experiencing any problems, no change in supplementation is required. However, you should be aware that it is not unusual to experience an exacerbation of existing symptoms or to develop flu-like symptoms for two or three days following an amalgam replacement appointment. Consequently, if after a week there has been a worsening of any existing symptoms or you experience new symptoms, you can make the following changes to the program. If you have experienced new symptoms not present prior to supplementation, they may be caused by either the supplement itself or the particular brand you are taking. (Most manufacturers use different types of fillers to meet FDA tablet size requirements). If you do feel it is the supplements, then stop taking everything and start retaking them one at a time for two or three day periods in an attempt to isolate the particular offender. If, however, the supplements have been well tolerated and the reaction has occurred only after amalgam replacement, try the following steps. If, after increasing dosages as indicated you experience an exacerbation of any symptomatology, stop taking all supplements and seek professional assistance.

1. Increase the glutathione to two capsules three times per day for a total of 6 capsules or 300 milligrams.

31

2. Increase vitamin C to 1,000 milligrams with each meal and 1,000 milligrams 1 hour after supper.

3. Add pantothenic acid. One 100 milligram tablet with breakfast and supper.

4. Add an amino acid complex. Mercury has the ability to deplete or impair utilization of several amino acids. Clinical experience of some physicians indicates that the addition of an amino acid complex has supplied the proper balance in intractable cases. Take one hour before meals or at bedtime.

If possible, detoxification should be started at least two weeks before scheduled amalgam removal/replacement and continued throughout the treatment plan. After completion of your dental treatment plan, continue on the detoxification protocols for an additional 30-60 days. You will be the best judge, based on how you are feeling, as to when to reduce, modify, or stop the supplements.

As stated elsewhere in this book, detoxification is more than just taking supplements. Dietary and lifestyle modifications are an essential adjunct to supplementation. In this regard, please pay special attention to the information contained in Appendix B, which explains the benefits of a high-fibre diet as an integral part of your detoxification process. Additionally you should give up chewing gum until all the mercury amalgam fillings have been replaced. If possible, weekly sweat therapy should be instituted at the same time as supplementation. Sweat therapy does not mandate steam baths or saunas. Any exercise or activity that causes sweating serves the desired purpose of inducing the excretion of toxins and heavy metals through the skin. Regardless of the modality used, the objective should be to participate in the sweat generating activity for at least 30 minutes per session.

NOTE: Pregnant women and individuals with high blood pressure or heart disease should obtain approval from their physician before initiating sweat therapy.

For those individuals who have a great deal of trouble staying on a program, there is a product on the market that may provide you with a comparatively simple solution. Recently, a product called UltraClear® has been demonstrated to be effective in providing essential nutritional support during mercury detoxification following amalgam replacement. UltraClear® can only be obtained from a health care professional and utilized under their direction. UltraClear® is a therapeutic food composed of white rice protein concentrate, medium-chain triglycerides, high molecular weight rice dextrins, and mercury-detoxifying nutrients including ascorbate, glutathione, selenomethionine, and N-acetylcysteine. It is a 7-21 day program and patients whose amalgams have been replaced take UltraClear three to five times per day as a beverage, along with foods specified in the Ultra Clear metabolic detoxification program booklet. If your health care professional is not using the program, you can possibly get the name of a health care professional near you administering the UltraClear program, by contacting HealthComm, Inc., (800) 843-9660.

DENTAL OFFICE PROTOCOLS

The last point we would like to make concerns the proper protocols for the removal of mercury amalgam dental fillings. Try to locate a dentist who knows about protecting his patients from mercury and does not place mercury fillings, (mercury-free). Some people react to the levels of mercury vapor at the dentist's office.

There are special techniques utilized by your dentist to remove mercury amalgam fillings. If done properly, there is minimum exposure to increased levels of mercury vapor caused by the removal procedure. However, we feel it important that you should be aware of certain aspects related to removing mercury from the oral environment:

The office and operatory should be well-ventilated.

The dentist should have an assistant present to assist in minimizing their exposure, and yours, to any mercury vapor. The correct protocol requires the use of high volumes of cold water both from the drill and separate irrigation by the assistant, who should also be simultaneously using high volume suction evacuation of the vapor and particles resulting from the removal procedure.(29) The requirement for copious amounts of cold water during amalgam removal is well documented and cannot be overly emphasized. Even dentists who are not mercury-free should know this. Failure of a dentist to be aware of this should be considered a sign of a lack of knowledge on the subject. Sadly, some dentists still drill out old amalgam with very little or even no water spray. Should you encounter a dentist who is unaware or inattentive to this, you would be well advised to seek treatment elsewhere.

It is the volatility of mercury that necessitates all the precautions and correct techniques. Mercury vapor pressure doubles with every ten degree centigrade rise in temperature. One acceptable procedure that minimizes extensive grinding (which generates great temperature increases) involves sectioning the amalgam into chunks versus just grinding it out.

In some dental offices the dentist may ask you to breathe through a nose piece that will permit you to draw air from another area of the operatory or office. If the dentist has nitrous oxide/oxygen available and you have elected to use it, this will accomplish the same thing.

The use of the rubber dam during the amalgam removal procedure is still controversial at this time. Some believe it to be essential, while others maintain that it results in amalgam particles and mercury vapor being trapped under the dam during the entire procedure. These latter contend that careful attention to removal and evacuation results in lower mercury exposure to the patient.

Clean Up^{TM} is a recently developed new type of oral aspirator/evacuator product from Sweden that is now available in the United States. The Clean Up device fits over the tooth being worked and applies a constant suction to the immediate work area, thereby greatly reducing extra-oral aerosol spray and possible infectious particulate. Clean Up^{TM} is available in the United States from Future Dentistry, Inc. (800)-282-9670

During the procedure, the dentist and his assistant are at greater risk to mercury vapor exposure than the patient. To protect themselves, they will be putting on special mercury trapping masks and rubber gloves to protect them during repeated removal operations.

Don't be in a hurry. Current information indicates that it is better to replace only a few amalgams at a time, with several weeks in between appointments.

Unless your physician or dentist has deemed it absolutely essential and critical to a diagnosis, do not permit x-rays of any kind to be taken during pregnancy. If dental x-rays are deemed essential, do not permit them to be taken unless a lead apron of suitable size is utilized to cover the area from the chin down over the abdomen. There is substantial scientific documentation demonstrating the toxic maternal and fetal effects from extremely low-dose radiation.(30-31)

One question related to amalgam replacement that we get a great number of calls on deals with a protocol called "sequential removal." Sequential removal requires the dentist to measure and chart the electrical current of each filling and to remove/and or replace the amalgam fillings based on the charted information, starting with the highest negative readings first. There is no scientific data to support the use of sequential removal. Additionally, there is absolutely no scientific data to support the statements being made by the proponents of sequential removal that "if your dentist doesn't use sequential removal it will cause the mercury to be locked into the tissues." It has been well established scientifically that precise measurement of these electrical currents or comparison of the electrical currents emanating from various amalgams is not possible. Amalgam is an unstable material to start with and measurements are of specific points on the filling, not the entire filling. Therefore, they cannot be compared to each other. The simple truth is that most dentists around the world are replacing amalgam fillings with nonmetallic fillings by quadrant, usually starting with the quadrant that has the largest fillings, thus removing the largest source of mercury first. The results achieved with removal by sequential removal cannot be distinguished from those achieved with quadrant removal. Therefore, if your dentist has the equipment and wants to replace your amalgam fillings sequentially, there is no problem in allowing it. Just bear in mind that it is not a prerequisite for successful amalgam filling replacement.

DETOXIFICATION UTILIZING DRUGS

Acute or other diagnosed cases of mercury intoxication are treated by the toxicologist/physician by using metal binding drugs that have been approved by the FDA. The most common of these dates back to World War II where it was originally developed as an antidote to "lewisite", an arsenical war gas. The British found that thiol compounds could successfully compete with the tissue SH groups for the arsenicals. The most effective was a dithiol compound that was named Dimercaprol, also commonly referred to as BAL, which is the acronym for British Anti-Lewisite. After the war it was discovered that Dimercaprol was effective against other heavy metals, including mercury. Like most drugs, Dimercaprol does have side effects which we feel are significant enough that you should request your physician to use or prescribe something else. It is lipid-soluble, enters cells and inactivates many enzymes. Actually, it increases mercury levels in the brain. Another drug used for mercury detoxification is D-Penicillamine. Both drugs utilize the affinity of mercury for the sulfur molecule as the basis of their therapeutic effectiveness. Dimercaprol must be administered by injection but D-Penicillamine is well absorbed from the gut and can be given orally and is less toxic.(32,33)

DMPS (2,3-Dimercapto-1-Propanesulfonic Acid) is a water-soluble derivative of Dimercaprol developed to reduce the side effects of Dimercaprol and is marketed in countries outside the U.S. under the brand name Dimaval[TM]. DMPS can be given orally and appears to have few serious side effects. It has been used effectively in Russia since 1957 where it is known as Unithiol. Another important orally administered antidote for heavy metal poisoning is DMSA (2,3-Dimercaptosuccinic Acid) which has been studied extensively by the Chinese, Russians and Japanese since 1957. A major difference between DMSA and DMPS is that DMSA accelerated mercury elimination from the brain, but DMPS had no effect, and mercury levels in the blood, kidneys and liver were decreased more effectively by DMSA.(34,35) The FDA has recently approved DMSA for use in the United States for the treatment of childhood lead intoxication. The product name is Chemet[TM], marketed by McNeil Pharmaceuticals.

Unithiol is used as a diagnostic tool in the Soviet Union. Urinary mercury levels which increase more than 8 times after Unithiol administration, together with symptoms of poisoning, is indicative of poisoning. Heyl Co., German manufacturer of Dimaval[TM] recommends an oral dosage of 300-400 milligrams per day in divided doses. Heyl also has a 250 mg injectable preparation of Dimaval which Max Daunderer, M.D., a toxicologist in Munich, Germany, has used to successfully treat over 800 amalgam/mercury toxic patients.(35) Many of his patients who had replaced their amalgam dental fillings years previously but who still exhibited many symptoms of mercury poisoning, dumped large quantities of mercury in their urine after iv Dimaval. There was a subsequent amelioration of symptomatology after Dimaval. Dr. Daunderer's clinical experience indicates that the first weeks after treatment there will usually be a worsening of symptoms with an immediate metal taste, tiredness, dizziness and then an improvement. In many instances the excreted amounts of mercury are not exceptionally high. It is our understanding that the Heyl Co. is testing and collecting data on DMPS in the United States, as a requirement of FDA approval for its use in this country.

Dr. Hanson (Sweden) believes that Dimaval can be used to decrease any adverse effects during amalgam removal and recommends that neurological patients should have immediate treatment (ALS, MS). We are also aware of DMSA being used very effectively for the same purpose during amalgam removal. The availability of DMSA in the U.S. dictates that serious consideration be given to its use during amalgam removal for all patients with neurological problems.

DMPS is a very safe drug which has even been used to treat lead poisoning in 3-5 year old children without any side effects. DMSA is even less toxic. DMSA is taken orally 10-30 milligrams per kilogram of body weight. Many amalgam patients will have large deposits of mercury in the jaw bone. Large pieces of amalgam (even droplets of mercury) can only be removed by surgery but diffusely spread mercury can only be extracted chemically. In this regard, the Unithiols have been shown to be more effective than any other chelator. To remove mercury from tissues, the chelator must bind mercury more strongly than any substance already present in the body. In addition, the chelator must not remove metals from enzymes which require them to function properly. One word of caution about the use of DMPS and DMSA; they will also remove zinc. Zinc deficiency should be corrected prior to starting any chelator treatments and zinc should be supplemented during treatments.(36)

DETOXIFICATION USING HOMEOPATHIC REMEDIES

The basic philosophy underlying homeopathy is that 'like cures like.' In other words if you are suffering a particular set of symptoms, you normally would be given a homeopathic remedy that induces the same symptoms. This procedure activates and stimulates the body's natural defenses in the same manner as do immunization shots to protect against certain diseases - a well accepted procedure. Be assured there is nothing simple about homeopathy. To use it properly requires a great amount of training on the part of your health provider. There is one thing that can be said for homeopathy and that is that in the hands of a skilled practitioner - it works. The practice of homeopathy has been well established in Europe for scores of years and is gaining renewed favor in the United States. However, a word of caution is in order. Verify the credentials of anyone who wants to prescribe homeopathic remedies for you and make sure that he is either Boarded or has taken extensive training from reputable sources. [The National Center for Homeopathy; 801 North Fairfax Street; Alexandria, Virginia 22314, telephone (703) 548-7790 may be able to provide you with the name of a physician or dentist in your area trained in homeopathy.]

DETOXIFICATION USING INTRAVENOUS EDTA.

Physicians who are members of the American College of Advancement in Medicine utilize intravenous EDTA to do heavy/toxic metal detoxification. This form of detoxification is very effective for reducing body burdens of a great many of the toxic metals, especially lead. Although the scientific literature indicates that mercury is not one of the toxic metals for which EDTA has a great binding affinity, some clinical experience and results indicate that additional mercury is excreted in the urine. For whatever reason, i.e., the tissue redistribution phenomenon that occurs during detoxification or EDTA binding with extra-cellular mercury, urine mercury levels appear to be higher after EDTA therapy. (EDTA is the abbreviation for ethylene-diamine-tetra-acetic acid which is an FDA approved synthetic amino acid.) Recently published research has shed a little more light on EDTA and mercury. EDTA removes mercury from cell surfaces

39

and in the blood but not from inside the cells. However, the attachment of mercury to EDTA is weak. [Write the American College of Advancement in Medicine; 23121 Verbugo Dr., Suite 204; Laguna Hills, CA 92653; or call 714-583-7666 to see if there is a physician available, in your area certified in intravenous EDTA detoxification]

LET YOUR VOICE BE HEARD

There has always been a very small minority of the individuals that have undergone amalgam replacement that have not benefited from it. This has caused a great deal of discouragement in the individual and the health professional working with them. In some instances it has been related to the materials and procedures used by the dentist that did the work. In others it was assumed that their health problems were caused by something other than mercury or that the damage caused by mercury was irreversible. Whatever the reason, it was very little comfort to the individual not seeing any improvement. Now however, thanks to some very advanced research in Sweden, it appears there may be an answer for many of these intractable cases. Dr. Christer Malmström in Sweden has discovered that most of the people who do not see health improvements after amalgam replacement appear to have diverticula or impacted fecal matter in their colon that contains high levels of toxic metals. Upon removal of these metals, great progress can be seen in the individual's health. Appendix B contains a complete review of Dr. Malmström's protocol.

Even in those cases where there hasn't been any great improvement, these individuals can take comfort from the fact that they have eliminated a constant source of poison entering their body. The vast majority of individuals who have undergone amalgam replacement and the reduction of their mercury body burden have experienced improvements in health that have ranged from minor to startlingly dramatic. For example the statistics listed below were compiled by the Foundation For Toxic Free Dentistry (FTFD) on **1569** patients from 6 different reports:

% of Total	SYMPTOM	Total No.	No. Improved or Cured	% of Cure or Improvement
14%	ALLERGY	221	196	89%
5%	ANXIETY	86	80	93%
5%	BAD TEMPER	81	68	89%
6%	BLOATING	88	70	88%
6%	BLOOD PRESSURE PROBLEMS	99	53	54%
5%	CHEST PAINS	79	69	87%
22%	DEPRESSION	347	315	91%
22%	DIZZINESS	343	301	88%
45%	FATIGUE	705	603	86%
15%	GASTROINTESTINAL PROBLEMS	231	192	83%
8%	GUM PROBLEMS	129	121	94%
34%	HEADACHES	531	460	87%
3%	MIGRAINE HEADACHES	45	39	87%
12%	INSOMNIA	187	146	78%
10%	IRREGULAR HEARTBEAT	159	139	87%
8%	IRRITABILITY	132	119	90%
17%	LACK OF CONCENTRATION	270	216	80%
6%	LACK OF ENERGY	91	88	97%
17%	MEMORY LOSS	265	193	73%
17%	METALLIC TASTE	260	247	95%
7%	MULTIPLE SCLEROSIS	113	86	76%
8%	MUSCLE TREMOR	126	104	83%
10%	NERVOUSNESS	158	131	83%
8%	NUMBNESS ANYWHERE	118	97	82%
20%	SKIN DISTURBANCES	310	251	81%
9%	SORE THROAT	149	128	86%
6%	TACHYCARDIA	97	68	70%
4%	THYROID PROBLEMS	56	44	79%
12%	ULCERS & SORES (ORAL CAVITY)	189	162	86%
7%	URINARY TRACT PROBLEMS	115	87	76%
29%	VISION PROBLEMS	462	289	63%

The above statistics involve a total of 1569 patients in six different studies: 762 patients utilized the FTFD Patient Adverse Reaction Report (see page 59) to individually report changes in their health directly to the FDA and the FTFD; Dr. Mats Hanson, Ph.D. reported on 519 Swedish patients; Henrik Lichtenberg, D.D.S. of Denmark reported on 100 patients; Pierre LaRose, D.D.S. of Canada reported on 80 patients; Robert L. Siblerud O.D., M.S. reported on 86 patients in Colorado as partial fulfillment of a Ph.D. requirement; and Albert V. Zamm, M.D., FACA, FACP reported on 22 of his patients.

One extremely interesting statistic relates to the incidence of allergies reported above. The recent January 1993 Public Health Service Report on Dental Amalgam states: "Only a small proportion of mercury-sensitized individuals respond adversely to the placement of amalgam restorations. The few case reports of adverse allergic reactions to amalgam involve skin reactions, such as rashes and eczematous lesions..."(37) The ADA maintains that the incidence of allergic reaction to amalgam dental fillings is extremely rare, with only 50 case histories being reported in the literature. Statements of this nature totally ignore valid peer reviewed scientific studies demonstrating an allergic reaction to dental amalgam ranging from 16.5% for non-allergic patients to 44% for fourth year dental students.(38-39) More importantly, as this symptom analysis demonstrates, the question is not whether the patient is allergic to dental amalgam but rather the direct causal relationship of mercury/amalgam dental fillings to the development of allergies to food, chemicals, and environmental factors.

In the above FTFD analysis, this is supported by the fact that 14% of the individuals reported some type of allergy and that after replacement of their mercury/amalgam dental fillings, 89% reported their condition had improved or was totally eliminated. If you were to extrapolate this data to the approximately 140 million amalgam bearers in the United States, there should be 19.6 million people (14%) with amalgam causally related allergies. Of this number, 89% or approximately 17.4 million would have their allergies ameliorate or disappear simply by having their mercury dental fillings exchanged for non-mercury ones.

We attempted to look at this from another perspective, by first determining the total number of people in the U.S. with allergies. Although there are no hard data available, the NIH estimates the number to be between 40-50 million. Using the lesser number of 40 million people with allergies, it is estimated that 65% (40) or 26 million of them would be amalgam bearers whose allergies may be causally related to their mercury/amalgam dental fillings. HARDLY AN INSIGNIFICANT NUMBER!

In democratic societies throughout the world, when the voices of the citizenry are raised in angry protest, the politicians and government usually respond in direct proportion to the degree of furor. It is a fact of life, pure and simple. It doesn't matter how long the problem or condition that provoked the people has been treated with benign neglect. When enough people express their concern, it is a clarion call to remedial action.

Thanks to the CBS "60 Minutes" Program on the amalgam issue that aired on December 16, 1990 and the great number of articles on the subject that appeared in major newspapers all across the country, millions of citizens of our country are now aware that a controversy exists on the continued use of mercury in dentistry. More and more people are insisting that no more mercury be placed in their teeth and are opting for alternative materials.

What is needed now is to let your voices be heard by your elected representatives, dentists, and physicians. Demand answers as to how the professional associations and governmental agencies involved have permitted mercury, an insidious poison, to be implanted in your body without your knowledge or consent. Demand that the U.S. government ban the use of mercury in dentistry, all pharmaceuticals whether prescription or nonprescription, and its use in cosmetics, without further delay. Additionally, the Congress must insure that medical and dental insurers make adequate provisions to reimburse individuals who have had their mercury dental fillings replaced for medical reasons.

REFERENCES

1. Dorland's Illustrated Medical Dictionary, 25th Edition, 1974. W.B. Saunders Co., Philadelphia.
2. An Assessment of Mercury in the Environment. National Academy of Sciences. Washington, D.C., 1978.
3. Clarkson T.W., Friberg L., Hursh J.B. and Nylander M. The prediction of intake of mercury vapor from amalgams, pp 247-264. In: Biological Monitoring of Toxic Metals. Plenum Press. New York, Feb 1988.
4. Environmental Health Criteria 118: Inorganic Mercury. World Health Organization, International Programme on Chemical Safety (IPCS), 1991 Geneva, Switzerland.
5. Arvidson K. Corrosion studies of a dental gold alloy in contact with amalgam under different conditions. Swed Dent J 68:135-139, 1984.
6. Skinner EW. The Science of Dental Materials. 4th Edition revised. W.B. Saunders co. Philadelphia pp 284-285, 1957.
7. Clarkson T.W. (Chairman) Mercury Health Effects Update.- Health Issue Assessment. U.S. Environmental Protection Agency. EPA-600/8-84-019F, August 1984. Final Report.
8. Ziff S., and Ziff M.F. Infertility & Birth Defects. Is Mercury From Silver Dental Fillings an Unsuspected Cause? Bio-Probe, Inc. Orlando, FL Dec 1987.
9. Braverman, E.R. and Pfeiffer C.C. The Healing Nutrients Within: Facts, Findings and New Research on Amino Acids. Keats Publishing, Inc. New Canaan, CT. 1987.
10. Flanagan RJ., Meredith TJ. Use of N-Acetylcysteine in clinical toxicology. The Am J of Med. 91 (suppl 3C):131S-139S, Sept 30, 1991.
11.. Livardjani F. et al. Lung and blood superoxide dismutase activity in mercury vapor exposed rats. Toxicology 66:289-295, 1991.
12. Girardi G., Elias MM. Effectiveness of N-acetylcysteine in protecting against mercuric chloride-induced nephrotoxicity. Toxicology 67:155-164, 1991.
13. Nutra Letter. Faulty Sulfur Metabolism Linked to Allergic Illness. Vol 4(1):1-4, August 1990
14. Moeschlin S. (Ed), Klinik und Therapie der Vergiftungen. 6th edition. 1980. G. Threme, Verlag.
15. Pfeiffer C.C. Mental and Elemental Nutrients, pp 139-140, 1975. Keats Publishing, New Canaan, CT.
16. Rowland I.R. et al. The effect of various dietary fibers on tissue concentration and chemical form of mercury after methylmercury exposure in mice. Arch Toxicol. 59(2):94-98, 1986.
17. Summers A.O. et al. Increased mercury resistance in monkey gingival and intestinal bacterial flora after placement of dental "silver" fillings. The Physiologists, September 15, 1990
18 Anderson J.W., et al. Hypocholesterolemic effects of oat-bran or bean intake for hypercholesterolemic men. American Journal of Clinical Nutrition. 40:1146-1155, 1984.
19. Katsunuma T. et al. Exercise-induced anaphylaxis: Improvement after removal of amalgam in dental caries. Ann Allergy 64:472-5, May 1990.
20. Vimy M.J., Takahashi Y., and Lorscheider F.L. Maternal-fetal distribution of mercury (^{203}Hg) released from dental amalgam fillings. Am J. Physiol. 258 (Regulatory Integrative Comp. Physiol. 27):R939-R945, 1990.

22. Beach R.S., Gershwin M.E., and Hurley L.S. Persistent immunological consequences of gestation zinc deprivation. Am J Clin Nutr. 38:579-590, October 1983.

23. Beach R.S., Gershwin M.E., and Hurley L.S. Gestational zinc deprivation in mice: Persistence of immunodeficiency for three generations. Science. 218: 469-470, October 1982.

24. Quirin H. Pain and Viatamin B1 therapy. Bibl Nutr Dieta 38:110-111, 1986.

25. Blakley BR. et al. The effects of thiamine on tissue distribution of lead. J Appl Toxicol. 10(2):93-97, 1990.

26. Lieberman s. and Bruning N. The Real Vitamin & Mineral Book. pages 63-69, 1990. Avery Publishing Group.

27. Kamen B. B vitamins from acidophilus. page 28, Health World, March-April, 1990.

28. Miller JM. et al. The administration of bromelain orally in the treatment of inflammation and edema. Exp Med Surg. 22:293-299, 1964.

29. Richards J.M. and Warren P.J. Mercury vapor released during the removal of old amalgam restorations. Br. Dent J. 159(7): 231-232, 1985.

30. Hobbs C.H. and McClellan R.O. Chapter 21: Toxic effects of radiation and radioactive materials. pp 669-705. In, Caserett and Doull's Toxicology (3rd ed). Macmillan Publishing Co. NY, 1986.

31. Norwood C. At Highest Risk. Protecting Children From Environmental Injury. Chapter 6, pp 156-188, Penguin Books. 1981.

32. Goyer R.A. Chapter 19: Toxic Effects of Metals. pp 582-635. In: Caserett and Doull's Toxicology (3rd ed). Macmillan Publishing Co. NY, 1986.

33. Klaassen C.D. Chapter 69: Heavy Metals and Heavy-Metal Antagonists. pp 1615-1637. In: Goodman and Gilman's The Pharmacological Basis of Therapeutics (6th ed). Macmillan Publishing Co. NY, 1980.

34. Aposhian H.V. DMSA and DMPS - water soluble antidotes for heavy metal poisoning. Ann Rev Pharmacol Toxicol 23:193-215, 1983.

35. Daunderer M. Mobilization test for environmental metal poisonings. Forum des Praktischen und Allgemdn-Arztes 28(3):88, 1989. English translation in the Bio-Probe Newsletter, 5(6):5-10, November 1989.

36. Flora SJ, Tandon SK. Beneficial effects of zinc supplementation during chelation treatment of lead intoxication in rats. Toxicology 64(2):129-139, Nov 1990.

37. DENTAL AMALGAM: A Scientific Review and Recommended Public Health Service Strategy for Research, Education and Regulation. Final report of the subcommittee on risk management of the committee to coordinate environmental health and related programs public health service. Department of Health and Human Services January 1993.

38. Djerassi E. and Berova N. The possibilities of allergic reactions from silver amalgam restorations. Int Dent J 19(4): 481-488, 1969.

39. Miller EG, Perry WL, and Wagner MJ. Prevalence of mercury hypersensitivity in dental students. J Prosthetic Dent. 58(2):235-237, August 1987.

40. Dental Mercury - An Environmental Hazard! Bio-Probe Newsletter. Volume 8, Issue 5, September 1992.

APPENDIX A.
A SIMPLE SELF-TEST FOR ZINC DEFICIENCY

Blood levels of zinc tend to stay "normal" until a pronounced deficiency has developed and subnormal tissue levels might correspond to blood levels that are within "normal" range. A test that reveals whether a physiological process, dependent on zinc, works properly is preferable.

A British chemist and zinc specialist, Dr. Bryce-Smith, has devised a simple test, based on the fact that taste recognition depends on zinc levels. Zinc, as you may know from experience, has a very distinctive taste. If you have zinc on your tongue, you know it right away. If instead, you are suffering from a zinc deficiency, the typical taste reaction will be diminished, delayed, or not be there at all.

The zinc taste test is simple and easy to self-administer.

There are liquid zinc products on the market specifically formulated for the zinc taste test. They may be purchased at most health food stores or mail order vitamin companies that carry mostly name brands. Or, if you wish, you can make up your own solution by mixing 100 milligrams of zinc sulfate powder in 100 milliliters of water. Make it up fresh in a plastic or glass container and use it promptly as it will lose its efficacy in a short time.

Take a teaspoon of the liquid solution into your mouth without swallowing. If you experience a "furry," unpleasant taste immediately or within 5-10 seconds, your zinc status is adequate. If you do not get the distinctive zinc taste within a minute but instead perceive only a taste like water, you have a pronounced zinc deficiency. Anything in-between will indicate good to low zinc status and the need for supplementation.

Normally zinc is excreted in the urine. Low zinc levels in the urine indicate that your body does not get enough. Preliminary studies in connection with evaluation of DMPS treatment of mercury poisoned patients show that low urinary levels of zinc correspond to inability to taste the zinc solution or a long delay until the taste is noticed.

APPENDIX B
THE MALMSTRÖM HIGH FIBER PROTOCOL

Recently we had the pleasure of talking with two practicing dentists from Sweden who also do extensive research. Over the years Dr's. Christer and Ingegerd Malmström have developed very specific protocols for amalgam replacement, based on their clinical and patient experiences. The protocol evolved from their study of those patients that show no improvement in their symptomatology after amalgam replacement. They have found that a number of individuals that did not get better had diverticula and also areas of the colon that were coated with hardened or impacted fecal matter that contained trapped particles of amalgam/mercury and other heavy metals. The discovery occurred when one such patient excreted large particles of amalgam/mercury after undergoing a barium enema x-ray study. As a consequence, those individuals that do not improve after amalgam replacement are requested to clean their intestinal tract through use of life style modification, dietary changes insuring adequate high fiber intake and even the use of fiber supplements such as those containing psyllium seed and guar. It was observed that most patients started to show important health improvements within two-three weeks of being on a high fiber diet.

As a result of their experiences with the non-improvement-after-replacement individuals, the Malmströms have developed the following protocol for working with patients that desire to have their amalgam fillings replaced with non-mercury containing materials:

Three weeks before initial appointment all patients must go on a high fiber diet consisting primarily of fruits, vegetables and legumes (beans, peas, etc.). This means eliminating most meat, fish and fowl from the diet.

In addition, the patient must stop smoking, stop the use of all drugs that are not absolutely necessary, stop birth control pills, remove any IUD device (to eliminate a

47

constant source of copper), eliminate coffee or caffeine, and take no iron supplementation of any kind, including those vitamins that may have iron contained as a part of the enteric coating of the tablet. Clinical observation of the efficacy of this pre-removal program has been that most people with various pre-existing health conditions show improvement in their health prior to their first appointment for amalgam removal. Again, based on clinical experience, patients who are constipated are required to have the condition corrected before they can receive dental treatment. This is based on the need for the body to actively excrete toxins after dental treatment involving amalgam/mercury and to help eliminate the possibility of amalgam/mercury particulate being incorporated into diverticula or any impacted colon fecal matter.

At the patient's appointment for amalgam replacement, they are given activated charcoal tablets to take immediately prior to treatment. During actual operative procedures removing amalgam, rinsing and aspirating the work area and mouth every 20 seconds is recommended. Since coming on the market, the Malmströms utilize the Swedish aspirating device called Clean Up^{TM}, which has eliminated the need for a special rinsing and aspirating every 20 seconds. The Malmströms have found that using this protocol, 80% of their patients do not experience any post-operative adverse reactions. Those individuals that experience any type of adverse reaction are requested to come back to the clinic. Based on their clinical history and the vitamin/mineral supplementation program they are on, recommendations are made to increase selected nutrients until the reaction ameliorates. Always conservative in their approach, initial appointments are restricted to replacing only one or two small amalgam fillings and observing the patient's reaction. The patient is required to call in if there is any type of adverse reaction and the patient is also called the evening of their first appointment to determine how they are doing.

Most mercury-free dentists have observed the phenomenon of those few individuals who do not obtain any significant improvement after they have eliminated their mercury implants and the constant source of dental mercury exposure. Traditionally, the emphasis relating to helping these individuals has been to increase nutrients that bind with mercury or counter its toxic effects. Now it appears that these individuals may be suffering from intestinal diverticula filled with fecal matter containing varying amounts of heavy metals that continue releasing their toxins.

The medical profession formerly treated diverticulosis by prescribing a bland, low fiber diet. Since scientific research has demonstrated that high fiber diets tend to cleanse and remove the impacted matter out of the diverticula, high fiber diets are now the recommended medical treatment for diverticulosis.(reference Merck Manual) NOTE: Individuals going on high fiber diets must do so slowly, especially anyone who is constipated. For example, if you are going to use bran cereal, start out with a 1/2 cup (about 9 gm of dietary fiber) and increase by increments until you have a satisfactory stool frequency and volume. If you are taking a fiber supplement the same philosophy applies, start out with a 1/2 teaspoon only. Whenever you increase roughage or bulk in your diet, you also must insure that you drink an adequate amount of fluid, six to eight glasses of water as a minimum. The major side effect of a high fiber diet will be increased flatus which tends to diminish as tolerance develops. In other words, don't be surprised if you have a lot of intestinal gas as a result of going on your high fiber diet, and don't let it deter you from staying on the high fiber diet. Anyone experiencing significant pain or rectal bleeding as a result of going on a high fiber diet should immediately contact their physician. Those individuals who have been experiencing chronic constipation for a number of years should consult with their physician and proceed to a high fiber diet only under your physicians direction.

APPENDIX C
PRE- AND POST-AMALGAM REPLACEMENT TESTING
TO ESTABLISH ACCEPTABLE DOCUMENTATION OF MERCURY BODY BURDEN RELATED TO THE PRESENCE OF AMALGAM DENTAL FILLINGS

Usually the immediate and primary goal of anyone who has been sick for any length of time is to just get better. Psychologically, the long suffering person is usually not interested in documenting the cause of their illness but rather only the "cure." It is not until after recovery from their health problems that they begin to dwell on the cause of their illness. Failure to take the time to document the cause of their previous illness or health condition frequently results in difficulty in obtaining insurance coverage for the procedures performed.

As a direct result of the many letters and conversations we have had with individual patients and dentists about this particular aspect of their treatment and recovery, we have elected to include a brief outline of the various tests that can be done to help document whether or not the amalgam dental fillings were in fact causally related to any health problems experienced.

The first criteria, of course, is that testing must be done prior to amalgam replacement and implementation of any detoxification protocols. This is necessary to establish a "base line" of values. Once a base line has been established for all the values to be monitored, then these values can be monitored by subsequent testing to determine whether changes that occur in the individual's health and base line values have any relationship to the elimination of mercury-containing dental fillings. Unfortunately, unless prescribed by a physician, most of the testing protocols we will describe will have to be paid for by the individual. These are all expenses that will be over and above those related to your dental treatment plan. However, they may serve as the basis for medical/dental insurance coverage and reimbursement by your insurance carrier.

ESTABLISHING YOUR INDIVIDUAL BASE LINE VALUES

1. Hair Analysis. This is a simple test that has been around for many years. However, it was not until recently that sufficient published research studies have clearly documented the validity of hair analysis for heavy metal screening. Although human hair primarily reflects organic mercury, studies have indicated that from 10-20% is inorganic mercury.(1) Regardless of composition, high mercury hair values, without any external source of exposure should be a matter of concern. A recent EPA report indicates that human hair is excellent for biological monitoring of mercury.(2)

2. Urine mercury, lead, copper, tin, and albumin. (The reason for taking lead levels is two-fold: 1) to rule out lead toxicity, or to show that the toxic effects of mercury are increased when lead is present. 2) Lead inhibits the enzyme delta-aminolevulinic acid dehydratase (ALA-D) and causes an increased excretion of delta-aminolevulinic acid (ALA). Mercury inhibits delta-aminolevulinic acid dehydrogenase, also identified as ALA-D.(3) If lead is not a factor but urine ALA-D is increased, then blood levels of ALA-D should be checked to see if either enzyme, dehydratase or dehydrogenase, has been inhibited, which would further tend to support the toxicity of the mercury body burden.

Copper, silver and tin are also given off by amalgam fillings. The presence of high copper, silver or tin in the urine could further indict amalgam fillings. Urine albumin may be indicative of mercury burden. The excretion of albumin is decreased during acute or chronic exposure to mercury. Research has shown an increase or normalization of urine albumin after replacement of amalgam fillings.

3. Urine mercury porphyrin profile. The testing of porphyrins is not new; what is new is that Dr. James Woods and his colleagues at the University of Washington at Seattle have refined the High Performance Liquid Chromatograph (HPLC) technique for the testing of porphyrins that can produce a profile specific to mercury.(3) In the near future, major diagnostic testing laboratories should be able to perform the special HLPC porphyrin profile.

51

4. Fecal metal screen. This is a single-sample, one-pass analysis of a stool specimen that provides information on 25 different elements. The feces is a major route of excretion for mercury and silver, yet it is a valid test that is seldom, if ever, performed to check for heavy metal body burden. Production and collection of this type of data would permit establishing correlations between the health condition of an individual, the numbers and surfaces of amalgam dental fillings and fecal content of mercury as well as other amalgam metals such as silver, copper, tin and zinc.(5)

As explained in Appendix B, fecal analysis also presents, a method of tracking and documenting an individuals progress towards better health. We have been unsuccessful in locating a certified laboratory in the U.S. with the necessary equipment, or the willingness, to do commercial fecal metal screens of multiple metals. One reason for this may be the tremendous cost and effort involved. For example, we have been advised that the instrumentation itself costs over five million dollars and that calibration of the instrument for validity of results can take two to three years. We consider the use of this type of analysis so important to the mercury intoxicated individual that we have established a working relationship with the laboratory in Sweden doing this type of analysis. The service will be made available through your dentist or physician. Anyone interested in securing a fecal analysis please have your dentist or physician contact Bio-Probe at (800) 282-9670 for more information.

5. Intra-oral mercury vapor levels, before stimulation by chewing gum for 10 minutes and after chewing gum for 10 minutes. The approved IAOMT intra-oral protocol should be utilized. This test is not diagnostic of mercury intoxication. What it will do, however, is provide an evaluation of how much mercury is being released from your amalgam dental fillings. The significance of this information is that science has clearly demonstrated that 80 to 100% of inhaled mercury vapor is absorbed from the lungs into the blood stream where it is then distributed throughout the body. From a documentation standpoint, intra-oral mercury vapor readings pre-amalgam removal

and post-amalgam removal will clearly document your exposure to mercury vapor from your amalgam dental fillings. NOTE: IAOMT approved protocols may be obtained from Phillip P. Sukel, D.D.S., FIAOMT, 1635 N. Arlington Heights Rd., Arlington Heights, IL 60004. (708) 253-0240.

6. Blood mercury levels. Whenever possible, any other blood base-lines desired should be done at the same time blood samples are taken to determine blood mercury levels. Although blood mercury levels are not diagnostic of chronic mercury toxicity, there is published research showing a decline in blood mercury levels after elimination of mercury-containing dental fillings.(6)

7. Saliva mercury, copper and tin levels. "No mercury has been detected in saliva samples unless there was a mercury vapor exposure. Salivary glands are primary organs of excretion of mercury, and excessive exposure to inorganic mercury can result in salivary gland enlargement as well as excessive salivation....Salivary mercury levels can be much higher than blood mercury levels...."(7)

8. MetaMetrix, Inc. has developed a test to determine functional liver detoxication capacity. Based on a caffeine challenge, saliva is evaluated for the disappearance of caffeine, which has been determined to be a direct indicator of cytochrome P-450 activity.(8) Because there is documented scientific information showing the inhibition of cytochrome P-450 by mercury, this particular test or other possible tests for cytochrome P-450 could be of major medical import in establishing what role, if any, mercury from mercury dental implants plays in the ability of the liver to detoxify xenobiotics.(9) In this regard, if post-replacement testing is done, it would confirm a change in cytochrome P-450 activity based solely on removing a chronic mercury exposure source.

9. Current scientific research is demonstrating that cysteine and glutathione status have a very definite influence on efficiency of immune function.(10-11) It could be of extreme significance to show a variation in blood and/or urine sulfur amino levels pre and post amalgam replacement.

MERCURY CHALLENGE OR MOBILIZATION TESTING.

After establishing a urine mercury base-line. It is extremely important to then subject the patient to a test that would have a bearing on demonstrating body burden. At the present time, science has established that approximately 80% of the mercury body burden is contained in the kidneys. The other 20% being distributed to the brain, other organs and glands. The express purpose of a challenge test, is to administer a chelating agent, that has been scientifically documented to bind mercury and cause its excretion from the body. Several are available. At the present time there are three FDA approved drugs that can be used for this purpose: British Anti-Lewisite (BAL), which is dimercaprol. Although effective and in use for more than 70 years, it does have many disagreeable and serious side-effects; Penicillamine has also been used by the medical profession for a great number of years and it too has many side-effects; 2-3 Dimercaprol succinic acid (DMSA) is the newest drug. It is a water soluble derivative of BAL that was approved by the FDA, in March of 1991, as a product to remove lead from children. However, it is also very effective for mercury and has minimal side effects.

The following protocol has been derived from the published literature and the *Physicians' Desk Reference*: Provide the patient with a prescription to purchase DMSA. Quantity of 100 mg capsules is determined by using 30 mg/kg of patient body weight, i.e., a 150 lb individual (75 kg) would require 75 x 30 = 2250 mg or 23 (100 mg) capsules. Provide the patient with a 24 hour urine collection kit and instructions for standard collection procedures (provided by the laboratory you intend to have do the analysis).

The DMSA is to be taken in three divided doses, 6 hours apart. All drugs, vitamins, minerals, amino acids should have been stopped for 24 hours prior to taking the DMSA and no supplements or drugs should be taken during the 24 hour period of urine collection. The decision regarding stopping any prescription medication for 48 hours to accomplish the Mobilization Test can only be done with written concurrence of a physician. Care must be taken not to contaminate the collection container. Starting at 6:00 A.M. take the first dose of DMSA. Collect the first urine starting at 8:00 A.M., and the patient must collect all urine voided for the next 24 hours. Take the 2nd dose of DMSA at noon and the 3rd dose at 6:00 P.M. Continue urine collection until 8:00 A.M. the following morning. Medication and any supplementation may begin again after completion of urine collection.

A mobilization blood sample should also be taken. The blood sample should be taken anytime between two and four hours after ingesting the first dose of DMSA (8:00 A.M.-10:00 A.M.). Samples should be assayed for mercury utilizing the same facility and procedure utilized to establish base-line blood mercury levels.

REFERENCES

1. Katz SA and Katz RB. Use of hair analysis for evaluating mercury intoxication of the human body: a review. J App Toxicol. 12(2):79-84, 1992.
2. Jenkins DW. Biological Monitoring of Toxic Trace Metals. Volume 1. Biological Monitoring and Surveillance. EPA-600/3-80-89. Pages 163-164, September 1980.
3. Woods J. et al. Quantitative Determination of Porphyrins in Rat and Human Urine and Evaluation of Urinary Porphyrin Profiles During Mercury and Lead Exposures. Lab Clin Med, 129(2):272-281, Aug 1992.
4. Homburger F; Hayes EW, Editors. A Guide To General Toxicology. Pages 233-235. Karger Continuing Education Series, Vol. 5. S. Karger AG, Switzerland. 1983.
5. Skare I and Engqvist A. Amalgam restorations - an important source to human exposure of mercury and silver. LÄKARTIDNIGEN 15:1299-1301, 1992. (English translation by authors available through Bio-Probe).
6. Snapp KR, Boyer DB, Peterson LC, and Svare CW. The contribution of dental amalgam to mercury in blood. J Dent Res 68(5):780-785, May, 1989.
7. Stoppford, W. Chapter 15, Industrial exposure to mercury, page 387, in The Biogeochemistry of Mercury in the Environment, J.O. Nriagu Editor. Elsevier/North-Holland Biomedical Press, New York, 1979.
8. Functional Liver Detoxication Capacity Analysis. MetaMetrix, Inc. Medical Laboratory. 5000 Peachtree Industrial Blvd., Suite 110, Norcross, Georgia 30071. J. Alexander Bralley, Ph.D. Laboratory Director. (404) 446-5483. FAX (404) 441-2237. Also see "Metabolic Detoxification and Managing the Chronically Ill Patient" by Jeffery Bland, Ph.D. HealthComm, Inc. P.O. Box 1729, Gig Harbor, WA 98335. (206) 851-3943 or (800) 843-9660.
9. Veltman JC. and Maines MD. Alterations of Heme, Cytochrome P-450, and Steroid Metabolism by Mercury in Rat Adrenal. Archives Biochem Biophys. 248 (2):467-478, 1986.
10. DeFlora S. et al. antioxidant activity and other mechanisms of thiols involved in chemoprevention of mutation and cancer. The Am J Med. 91(suppl 3C):122S-130S, Sept 30, 1991.
11. Eck HP et al. Low concentrations of acid-soluble thiol (cysteine) in the blood plasma of HIV-1 infected patients. Biol Chem Hoppe Seyler 370:101-108, 1989.

FOUNDATION FOR TOXIC FREE DENTISTRY

The Foundation For Toxic Free Dentistry has been established to fulfill several vital functions:

1. To gather accurate information on the health effects of materials used in dental treatment.

2. To distribute this information to its membership by means of a newsletter.

3. To assist in the distribution of this information to the general public.

4. To provide assistance in the legal defense of the right of the public to receive this information and the right of professionals to provide this information and allied services to their patients.

5. To gather and disseminate information on nutrition and diet in relation to oral health and disease.

6. To provide referrals to dentists (physicians whenever possible) familiar with the literature on mercury toxicity and who realize that amalgam dental fillings provide the greatest source of chronic exposure to mercury vapor and abraded amalgam particles.

The Foundation has been established as a not-for-profit organization, similar to a highly successful and influential group that has been in operation for a number of years in Sweden.

The Swedish group was organized to provide a support organization for those individuals who felt that they had been poisoned by their mercury amalgam dental fillings. This organization has been very effective in bringing the potential toxicity of mercury amalgam fillings to the attention of the Swedish media, public and the Swedish Parliament. The Foundation hopes to be just as effective in this country.

A number of potentially harmful materials are routinely used in the course of dental treatment. Dental materials that have been known to present possible health risks include: Mercury; nickel; beryllium; chrome; cobalt; copper; silver; fluoride; and radioactive uranium.

The use of these materials presents a unique threat in that they are routinely placed directly in the body, often for long periods of time. Furthermore, the environment in which they are placed, the oral cavity, is uniquely harsh and suitable for transfer of these materials into the body cells themselves.

A determined minority of scientists and professionals has focused attention on evidence that these materials may present significant health risks to patients. Worldwide, more and more research is appearing that casts significant doubt on the wisdom of using these materials for dental treatment.

There is more than sufficient evidence casting doubt on the safety of the mercury released from dental amalgam fillings to constitute a legitimate scientific issue. This fact notwithstanding, the American Dental Association is busy reaffirming the safety of dental amalgam. In fact, the entire dental establishment seems to be mobilizing their efforts and resources to brand as "quackery" or "fraud" any statements or actions contrary to their established policy of saying that it is perfectly safe to implant a poison in your body, except in those few rare instances when the individual may be allergic to the poison.

Do you have the right to know what materials are placed in your mouth? Do you have the right to know what possible effect they may have on your health or that of your children? Are you aware that the causes of many common disease states are not known by the medical profession? Did you know that exposure to heavy metals, particularly mercury vapor, can cause pathological damage that is indicative of many of these disease states?

Evidently, the American Dental Association does not believe that you have any of the rights outlined above because in June of 1987 they took the unprecedented action of inserting into their Principles of Ethics and Code of Professional Conduct, Section 1-J, a provision making it improper and unethical to remove amalgam restorations from the non-allergic patient for the alleged purpose of removing toxic substances from the body, when such treatment is performed solely at the recommendation or suggestion of the dentist. In effect, this limits your dentist from even mentioning the potential hazards of the mercury being constantly released from any silver mercury fillings that you may have.

It is the Foundation's position that this is a clear violation of the rights of both the patient and the doctor and a misguided attempt to suppress scientific and medical progress. There is an effort underway in some states to enact legislation that will permit physicians and dentists to practice alternative therapies and to also insure that the patient's right to information is not arbitrarily limited by special interest groups.

PATIENT ADVERSE REACTION REPORT.(PARR)

FTFD has developed a two-part form that is being used to report information to the U.S. Food and Drug Administration (FDA). Each patient who is having or has had their mercury-containing dental fillings replaced with non-mercury dental fillings should complete a PARR form. In their own words, the patient lists the major health problems or symptoms that existed prior to having their amalgam dental fillings exchanged for non-mercury containing fillings. Approximately six-months after the last filling has been replaced, the patient indicates on the form whether their condition improved, remained the same, or got worse. The original of the PARR form is sent to the FDA and the duplicate copy is forwarded to the FTFD. The FTFD has established a computer file for each form and every symptom or problem listed is entered along with the results of amalgam replacement. Statistics such as those displayed on page 41 are derived from the file. The FDA has also established a computer file on the PARR forms submitted to them. Anyone desiring a PARR form can have one by requesting it from FTFD.

DENTAL & HEALTH FACTS

The Foundation Newsletter "Dental & Health Facts" will provide supporters and the general public the latest information on dental materials and new techniques and procedures for their use. It will also provide nutritional information related to the oral environment considered to be of interest and concern to the members. Perhaps more importantly, it will on a national basis attempt to keep the membership abreast of all the legal and legislative information related to the basic issues.

MERCURY-FREE DENTIST REFERRAL SERVICE

One other major service the Foundation provides is referrals to mercury-free dentists. These are dentists who have indicated that they do not place mercury/amalgam dental fillings any longer. Moreover, these dentists have a true appreciation for the great amount of mercury vapor that can be generated during removal operations and use every precaution available to protect and minimize unnecessary patient and staff exposures. They should all have training and have extensive experience in the proper placement of alternative composite materials. Having said this, the reader must understand that neither the Foundation, nor the DAMS coordinators have personal knowledge of most of the dentists on their referral lists. Consequently, you must call and, by asking intelligent questions, determine if the dentist you have been referred to is acceptable to you. The first question of course is "Do you place amalgam fillings?" If the answer is yes, look for another dentist. If the answer is NO then you should be concerned with how long they have been mercury-free and their experience and training in the placement of composites.

For a free sample issue of the Foundation Newsletter, PARR form, or referral to the closest mercury-free dentist on their list, simply send your request to FTFD or FOUNDATION FOR TOXIC FREE DENTISTRY, P.O. BOX 608010, ORLANDO, FL 32860-8010. Please also include with your request a #10 self addressed and stamped envelope.

If you wish to join the Foundation, include a check or money order payable to FTFD or Foundation For Toxic Free Dentistry in the amount of $15.00 in U.S. funds. Membership applications from foreign countries (other than Canada) please add an additional $15.00 to cover the increased postage costs (total $30.00 U.S.).

The FTFD is staffed by all volunteer help and all monies collected are used only for approved FTFD projects. The Foundation For Toxic Free Dentistry is 501(c)(3)nonprofit tax-exempt organization. Your gifts are tax deductible to the full extent the law allows. Additional contributions are welcomed.

DENTAL AMALGAM MERCURY SYNDROME (DAMS)

Some very wonderful people, most of them prior victims of mercury poisoning from their mercury/amalgam dental fillings, have started forming victim support groups, most bearing the name DAMS. These individuals feel a strong obligation to their fellow citizens to inform them of the potential health hazards of inhaling mercury vapor and swallowing abraded particles of mercury from their amalgam dental fillings 24 hours a day, 365 days a year.

Although removal of mercury/amalgam dental fillings does not guarantee health improvements, as the FTFD analysis on page 41 indicates most people who have replaced their mercury fillings with gold or composite fillings have experienced reversal or improvement of persistent health problems. Many experienced these life-altering improvements after years of suffering and frustration without ever receiving a valid medical diagnosis or having the cause of their health problem identified.

That unfortunate situation stems from the fact that most physicians have been lulled, by the dental establishment, into believing that mercury released from amalgam dental fillings poses no threat to health except in those few people who may be allergic to it. Consequently, most physicians have never previously taken the patient very seriously when they asked "Can the mercury from my dental fillings be causing my health problems?" Science and clinical case histories are beginning to change that attitude.

There is a grass-roots movement across this country to require that every dental patient be given their constitutional right to FREEDOM OF CHOICE to say NO to mercury amalgam dental fillings for themselves and their loved ones; to promote the public's RIGHT TO KNOW the potential health hazards of constant daily exposure to mercury from mercury dental fillings and to ensure that concerned dentists have the right to inform their patients of this issue.

The dedicated individuals involved in the DAMS groups are all victims and all volunteers. They are trying to provide understanding and information to those individuals bewildered by their health conditions, and who are trying to gain additional knowledge about the potential health effects of mercury. DAMS coordinators may also be able to refer you to a mercury-free dentist in your area. It is important that you extend these people the courtesy of only writing to them initially if you are soliciting any information or help. There just aren't enough hours in the day for them to talk to everyone by telephone. The following is a partial listing:

» Murlene Brake, DAMS of New Mexico. 725-9 Tramway Lane, NE, Albuquerque, NM 87122. Murlene produces a National DAMS Newsletter which can be subscribed to for $15.00 per year. In addition, Murlene has become the primary focal point for information related to DAMS activities. To see if there is a DAMS Coordinator in your area, or to become active as a DAMS coordinator, please write to Murlene.

» Louise Herbeck, DAMS of Illinois. P.O. Box 9065, Downers Grove, IL 60515.

» Shirley Brown, DAMS of Colorado. P.O. Box 19032, Denver, CO 80209. Shirley produces a DAMS of Colorado Newsletter and accepts subscriptions at $15.00 per year.

» Robert O. Stephenson, DAMS of Alaska. 1837 No Way Lane, Fairbanks, AK 99079-6338.

» Caryolyn Smith, DAMS of Michigan. 426 Grant, Grand Haven, MI 49417.

» Marjorie Wells Lensgraf, Route 2, Hoff Lane, Knoxville, TN 37938

» Bernice Rudelick, 5608 Hillbrook Dr., Charlotte, NC 28226-8066.

» Carol Ward, 7426 Rhoads St., Philadelphia, PA 19151.

» Virginia Brown, P.O. Box 85156, Tuscon, AZ 85754-5156.

» Pat House, 10230 St. RD 38E, Lafayette, IN 47905

» Jude Sayce, P.O. Box 492, West Yarmouth, MA 02673

» Cheryl Quackenbush (This group is called ADAMS of Washington), P.O. Box 854 Kirkland, WA 98083-0854.

» **PLEASE CONTACT DAMS PEOPLE BY MAIL ONLY**